DSM–5 Transition Guide for

Contemporary Psychiatric–Mental Health Nursing

Third Edition

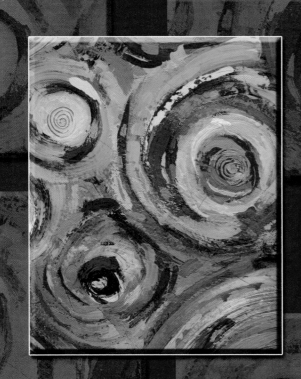

Carol Ren Kneisl
Eileen Trigoboff

PEARSON

Boston   Columbus   Indianapolis   New York   San Francisco   Upper Saddle River
Amsterdam   Cape Town   Dubai   London   Madrid   Milan   Munich   Paris   Montreal   Toronto
Delhi   Mexico City   São Paulo   Sydney   Hong Kong   Seoul   Singapore   Taipei   Tokyo

Cover and Title Page: shutterstock/fotoecho

V011
10 9 8 7 6 5 4 3 2

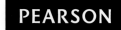

ISBN-10:   0-13-359730-X
ISBN-13: 978-0-13-359730-1

OUTLINE

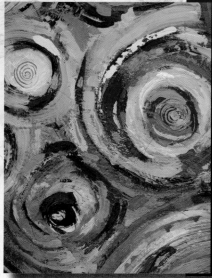

DSM-5 UPDATE FOR CONTEMPORARY PSYCHIATRIC– MENTAL HEALTH NURSING, 3/E

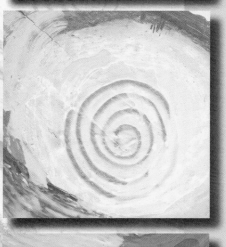

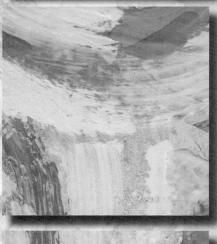

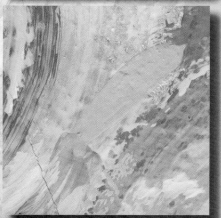

This module explains what you need to know about the relevant changes for psychiatric–mental health nursing practice from the *Diagnostic and Statistical Manual*, 4th Edition, Text Revision (DSM-IV-TR) to the *Diagnostic and Statistical Manual*, 5th Edition (DSM-5). We describe and review the major changes from DSM-IV-TR to DSM-5, including the diagnosis-specific changes (e.g., the revisions to the criteria for a diagnosis) and the broader, manual-wide changes (e.g., the use of dimensional assessments that cut across diagnostic categories, the integration of neuroscience research, and a broadened emphasis on development). We present rationales for why these changes took place so that you can better understand how the *Diagnostic and Statistical Manual* is best used in clinical practice. Minor revisions are summarized and the implications for nursing practice are listed. We organized this module to reflect the order of the chapters in our text, *Contemporary Psychiatric–Mental Health Nursing*, third edition, that discuss assessment, culture, mental disorders, and vulnerable populations. The table at the end of this module compares the features present in the DSM-IV-TR with the associated features now present in DSM-5, and their meaning for nursing practice.

There are several reasons why it is important to understand and use the DSM in clinical practice. One is that it provides you and other mental health professionals with a common language that minimizes confusion among the disciplines. By describing how mental disorders are expressed and how they can be recognized by mental health professionals, reliable diagnoses and appropriate treatment can be facilitated and a consensus in the mental health field created. Theoretically, by using the guidelines provided by the DSM, a psychiatrist in private practice in New York who has a biological orientation, a psychiatric–mental health nurse in primary care in Alabama who has an interpersonal orientation, and a psychologist in a state mental hospital in Kansas who has a behavioral orientation would all arrive at the same objective assessment and diagnosis of a client's symptoms.

The specifics that deal with changes in mental disorder categories are discussed in separate sections after this capsule view of the general changes:

- This version of the DSM is focused on accurately defining mental disorders that are significant in people's lives. It consists of a restructuring based on the disorders' apparent relatedness to one another, as reflected by similarities in underlying vulnerabilities and symptom characteristics.

- Chapters have been restructured to better reflect current scientific understanding of psychiatric disorders based upon new research in neuroscience and neuroimaging. The field trials that were the basis for the research and clinical application of the DSM tested the criteria for 23 disorders—15 adult and 8 child/adolescent diagnoses.

- The multiaxial system of the DSM-IV-TR has been replaced with a nonaxial documentation of diagnosis allowing for separate notations for psychosocial and contextual factors (formerly Axis IV) and for disability (formerly Axis V).

- Chapters are organized with a lifespan approach, that is, disorders most frequently diagnosed in childhood are at the beginning of the manual and disorders of older adulthood are at the end of the manual. Descriptions of how disorders may change across the lifespan are provided. There is no longer a separate chapter on children and adolescents.

- Severity is measured by a multidimensional set of severity scales that are clinically useful and simple to understand.

- Disorders that require further study, but are not yet sufficiently understood for routine clinical use, are discussed in a new section.

- Online supplemental information is available. Discussion of an electronic version (or e-version) of the DSM-5 has been vigorous. This would make it possible to update the manual as new information becomes available, making it unnecessary for users to wait a number of years between DSM revisions.

Health care professionals and mental health practitioners have begun to incorporate this version of the DSM-5 published in June 2013; however, full implementation is likely to evolve over a period of time. As new information becomes available through neurobiologic and sociologic research, further revisions are likely. For example, homosexuality was once a DSM mental disorder diagnosis in earlier versions of the manual until neurobiologic and sociologic research challenged the assumptions behind labeling homosexuality a mental disorder.

DSM-5 AND CHAPTER 9

CULTURAL COMPETENCE

The first official recognition of the role of culture in diagnosing mental illness appeared in Appendix I of the DSM-IV, which contained a Glossary of Culture-Bound Syndromes and an Outline of Cultural Formulation. The Appendix provided a method for categorizing and describing culture-bound disorders that paralleled, but did not precisely fit, DSM-defined disorders. The Glossary of Cultural Concepts of Distress serves that function in DSM-5.

The Cultural Formulation Interview (CFI), a new component, is a 16-item, structured, clinical interview to be administered during a client's initial assessment. The CFI is designed to make cultural formulation quicker and easier. Questions are designed to discover what exactly brought the client to seek help, the client's description of the problem and the stresses that make the problem worse. Family members and associates of the client may provide collateral information through the CFI Informant Version. It is unlikely that you will be asked to administer the CFI. This task falls to the professional carrying out the initial assessment. However, the information in the CFI can be used to enhance your nursing care plan for individual clients based on their culture.

Challenges to Clinical Practice

There is some concern among mental health professionals that while the CFI asks questions about cultural influences and interpretations, it does not differentiate content for specific cultures, nor does it provide guidelines to use when caring for clients from specific cultures. Because the cultural diversity of our communities continues to increase, clinicians will need to seek guidance for specific information about culture on an ongoing basis from resources other than the CFI.

DSM-5 AND CHAPTER 11

PSYCHIATRIC–MENTAL HEALTH ASSESSMENT

A new addition to the DSM is Section III Emerging Measures and Models with a segment on Assessment Measures. Because the DSM-5 recognizes the need for a dimensional diagnostic approach (one that cuts across categories of mental disorder), these measures are necessary for consistency. Psychiatric–mental health assessments routinely address the number and severity of an individual's symptoms in intensity, duration, and disability type(s). Hopefully, with further research, assessments will include more than subjective reports and clinical observations. A variety of objective measures such as reports on pathophysiology, gene/environment interactions, neurocircuitry functioning, and laboratory tests would be of great value. Cross-cutting symptom measures, severity measures, and the World Health Organization Disability Assessment Schedule 2.0 (WHODAS) make up assessment advances thus far.

Cross-cutting symptom measures are questions that help assess important areas of mental health. These areas (e.g., depression, anger, anxiety, memory, suicidal ideation) can be affected regardless of the psychiatric diagnosis. The individual client scores him- or herself according to a fairly straightforward scale, guiding clinicians toward areas that need further exploration. This is available as an adult self-report (which can also be used with children ages 11 to 17 with parent/guardian rating of symptoms). It can also be used by a knowledgeable adult informant for an impaired adult, and is available in child-rated versions.

The next addition to the assessment tools is the Clinician-Rated Dimensions of Psychosis Symptom Severity. This severity measurement, in the form of a rating-scale checklist, examines eight areas that give us information about how severe psychotic symptoms are. An example is: "Are hallucinations present but mild?" If this level of severity was chosen, it can be assumed that the client would not be very bothered by voices, or would not feel pressured to act. Each area has examples of the level of severity.

The World Health Organization Disability Assessment Schedule 2.0 (WHODAS) is a 36-item self-assessment measure that identifies levels of functioning in the past 30 days. Examples of the areas of disability include getting around and getting along with people.

Challenges to Clinical Practice

Being asked to complete self-assessments can be interpreted as a burden by many clients. If there is no informed and knowledgeable adult available to help the client with this task or to complete this information in the client's stead, then the dimensions of the diagnosis and the disability will not be fully explored.

DSM-5 AND CHAPTER 14

COGNITIVE DISORDERS

There has been an explosion of research in brain imaging, neuroscience, and neuropsychology in the past 20 years, resulting in several changes in our understanding of cognitive disorders. Dementia, delirium, amnestic, and other cognitive disorders are now referred to as Neurocognitive Disorders (NCDs). NCD is a broad category encompassing many symptoms and circumstances ranging from major to minor cognitive dysfunction. The diagnosis is now labeled in such a way as to attribute the problem to another process, such as Major Neurocognitive Disorder Due to Alzheimer's Disease. If there is uncertainty about the cause of the deficit, Probable and Possible indications are available. On the plus side, this category will also include people who have deficits in specific areas as a feature of HIV infection or traumatic brain injury, even at a young age. It prevents misdiagnosing a person who slips on cognitive tasks because of a stressor.

Challenges to Clinical Practice

What we see as a potential clinical problem is the possibility that everyday forgetfulness characteristic of advancing age could be diagnosed as Minor Neurocognitive Disorder (Frances, 2012). The presence of a diagnosis based on a symptom that could be explained by a number of nonpathologic processes may create a false-positive population of people who are not at special risk for a neurocognitive deficit. This label can create significant anxiety, even for those at true risk for developing dementia later. The possibility of a client being mislabeled in this regard could be emotionally damaging; therefore, caution regarding its use is encouraged.

Uncertainty of the cause of a neurocognitive deficit can be labeled as Probable or Possible and stated as emanating from, for example, Lewy Bodies. The problem arises when a clinician makes a judgment when the cause may not be clearly evident. Subsequent diagnostic and treatment decisions may possibly be based on a contamination or a bias in the direction of the original diagnostic statement.

DSM-5 AND CHAPTER 15

SUBSTANCE-RELATED DISORDERS

DSM-5 combines the categories of substance abuse and substance dependence in order to strengthen the diagnosis. Previous substance abuse criteria required only one symptom, whereas the DSM-5's mild substance use disorder category requires two to three symptoms.

Changes to DSM-5 affect the criteria used to assess alcohol problems. Overall, these changes will not likely change how often the diagnoses of alcohol problems are made, but may provide more precision in determining where someone is on the continuum of the problem. The more or less intensely the problem affects the client's functioning will be reflected in these refreshed standards for diagnosing. As alcoholism is a common disorder in our society, it will be important to explain to clients what these differences in the criteria and the diagnoses mean and to emphasize to the client that having difficulties three or four times a year still requires attention and treatment, even though on a different scale than would be necessary if one had problems with alcohol every weekend.

The addition of craving as a criterion for diagnosis could very well add a great deal to our understanding of the severity of alcohol problems.

Pathological Gambling, Cannabis Withdrawal, and Caffeine Withdrawal have been added to the substance-related disorders section.

Challenges to Clinical Practice

Because the changes involving diagnosis and craving result in categorizing individuals differently from how it has been in the past, there may be difficulty in comparing current and future research results with previous research outcomes. First-time substance abusers will be included in a diagnostic category with people who have had significant and dramatic, long-standing problems. Careful explanation would be necessary to define the different treatment needs and prognoses (Frances, 2012). It may also affect how people with this new diagnosis, Alcohol Use Disorder (AUD), accept and share their diagnosis, given the possibility of stigmatization.

One group of individuals who would have been previously diagnosed as abusing alcohol will no longer receive a diagnosis. These individuals tend to be male, belong to a higher socioeconomic group, and frequently exhibit driving under the influence as the only symptom of an alcohol problem. Because these individuals may no longer be eligible for treatment-related benefits, their well-being and the community's well-being should be carefully monitored (Edwards et al., 2013). These individuals could eventually progress to a diagnosis of Alcohol Use Disorder.

DSM-5 AND CHAPTER 16

SCHIZOPHRENIA

The newly coined category of Schizophrenia Spectrum and Other Psychotic Disorders in DSM-5 includes Schizotypal Personality Disorder. In DSM-5, Schizotypal Personality Disorder is considered to be within the schizophrenia spectrum (a small percentage of individuals go on to develop Schizophrenia) as well as a personality disorder. This is a divergence from previous conceptualizations in which personality disorders were distinctly different from the major mental disorders.

Attenuated Psychosis Syndrome (APS) is a new and controversial diagnosis included in the Other Specified Schizophrenia Spectrum and Other Psychotic Disorders category. This diagnosis does not meet the criteria for psychosis, as the person has insight and the symptoms are less severe and not as durable. In the process of using this particular diagnosis, a number of people could be diagnosed as having APS who would not otherwise be labeled thus. It is also a diagnosis listed as a condition for further study.

When one member of a relationship is delusional and the other individual does not meet the criteria for having Delusional Disorder but has some of the same beliefs, that second person can be given a diagnosis of Delusional Symptoms in Partner of Individual With Delusional Disorder. While this characterizes the weaker or less dominant of the pair as being psychologically vulnerable, having an actual diagnosis on the schizophrenia spectrum is a new feature. In DSM-IV, this was termed Shared Psychotic Disorder (*folie a deux*).

Challenges to Clinical Practice

While Schizotypal Personality Disorder is explored in DSM-5 in the personality disorder chapter, its inclusion in the schizophrenia spectrum is a conceptual shift. The challenge is to provide the distinctly different treatments for a disorder that is biologically based and requires neurotransmitter correction (or approximated correction) through pharmacology, and a distressing, interpersonal style that needs talk therapy.

A question raised by the diagnosis of Delusional Symptoms in Partner of Individual With Delusional Disorder is: How will services be accessed for people diagnosed with this disorder? Treatment would not likely be biologic, but psychosocial in nature.

With the conceptual shift in schizophrenia spectrum disorders, a challenge could be a drastic reduction in biologic treatment such as pharmacological agents, electroconvulsive therapy (ECT), and repetitive transcranial magnetic stimulation (rTMS). Research in antipsychotic agents and somatic treatment areas would be less likely to be funded and to occur. Current genetic-study results in schizophrenia would not apply to a continuum conceptualization. Our understanding of the process of psychosis would likely suffer as a result.

DSM-5 AND CHAPTER 17

MOOD DISORDERS

DSM-5 removes the bereavement exclusion in diagnosing mood disorders. In DSM-IV-TR this exclusion applied to people experiencing depressive symptoms lasting less than 2 months after the death of a loved one. DSM-5 distinguishes between grief and depression and recognizes that bereavement is a severe psychosocial stressor that can precipitate a major depressive episode beginning soon after the loss of a loved one (Frances, 2012). The exclusion has been removed and replaced by several notes within the text defining the differences between grief and depression. Therefore, an individual experiencing a grief reaction may well be diagnosed with a mood disorder.

Premenstrual Dysphoric Disorder (PMDD) has been moved from an Appendix in DSM-IV-TR to the diagnostic criteria and coding section of DSM-5. It is considered a depression associated with ovulation.

Disruptive Mood Dysregulation Disorder is a diagnosis for children who exhibit persistent irritability and frequent episodes of verbal or behavioral outbursts three or more times a week for more than a year. The diagnosis is intended to address concerns about potential overdiagnosis and overtreatment of bipolar disorder in children.

Challenges to Clinical Practice

An individual experiencing grief may well have a mood disorder triggered by a psychosocial event. It may be less likely that an individual would seek treatment during that difficult time in order to avoid being diagnosed and stigmatized. Treatment would essentially remain the same, although a psychiatric diagnosis could now accompany the loss. Normal grief will become Major Depressive Disorder, thus applying a medical/psychiatric diagnosis to our expected and necessary emotional reactions to the loss of a loved one and substituting pharmacology for the deep consolations of family, friends, spirituality, and the resiliency that comes with time and the acceptance of the limitations of life (Frances, 2012).

Premenstrual Dysphoric Disorder (PMDD) is now included in the main section on diagnostics and coding. This has been a controversial area; however, sufficient research now exists to characterize PMDD as a mental disorder.

Children in particular are the focus of the diagnosis of Disruptive Mood Dysregulation Disorder. The diagnosis of Bipolar Disorder in children had been heightened beyond the expected rate because in DSM-IV-TR there was no appropriate diagnosis for this cluster of symptoms in children. If children who have the diagnostic features of irritability for more than a year are reclassified as having a depressive Disruptive Mood Dysregulation instead of Bipolar Disorder, the rate returns to the expected level. Further exploration of this change is included in the Children and Adolescent chapter discussion.

DSM-5 AND CHAPTER 18

ANXIETY DISORDERS

Within the DSM chapter on anxiety disorders, the disorders are presented in the approximate order in which they would likely develop from childhood through adulthood. Generalized Anxiety Disorder is one of the diagnoses in this section that has had a number of small changes, but those changes can affect many in the population. For example, having everyday worries would be enough to justify an anxiety disorder diagnosis.

Obsessive-Compulsive Disorder and other related disorders have been separated from the Anxiety Disorders in DSM-5 and are now in a separate section. A new diagnostic category in this new section is Hoarding Disorder. It characterizes people who have a durable difficulty discarding or parting with possessions, regardless of the possession's actual or potential value. The behavior usually has harmful effects—emotional, physical, social, financial, and legal—for someone who hoards and for the family members. Recent research as well as media exposure to the phenomenon contributed to this new diagnosis. Excoriation (Skin-Picking) Disorder is another new diagnosis and is included in this section. Trichotillomania (Hair-Pulling Disorder) is also in this section.

Post-Traumatic Stress Disorder (PTSD), typically categorized as an anxiety disorder, is included in a new chapter in DSM-5 on Trauma- and Stressor-Related Disorders. The description of the syndrome focuses on the behavioral symptoms that accompany PTSD and has four distinct diagnostic clusters now, instead of the previous three. This specificity can be most useful in designing therapeutic approaches, both individual and group. With the increase in PTSD among military personnel, it is an important focus for all health care providers. The criteria for children and adolescents with PTSD has been expanded and detailed.

Challenges to Clinical Practice

Concern has been expressed in the literature about how the broader criteria for Generalized Anxiety Disorder pathologize the worries of everyday life. That is, the potential is heightened for creating new groups of people diagnosed with this anxiety disorder who otherwise may not have met the criteria presented in DSM-IV-TR. Medicating those individuals with antianxiety medications, a common treatment pathway, increases the risks for dependence and has not been proven to enhance positive outcomes (Frances, 2012).

While the PTSD criteria can be extraordinarily helpful in designing treatment programs, the chance of misdiagnosis in forensic settings could have important ramifications (Frances, 2012). The new manual includes a cautionary statement for forensic use of DSM-5. Claiming symptoms for secondary gain or to otherwise escape liability has always been an issue with a forensic population. The detailed expansion of included symptoms could offer a wider net within which people can hide.

It bears noting that the move of PTSD to a separate chapter, while acknowledging its place in the spectrum of trauma, may distract from its inherent anxiety-disorder roots. This has treatment implications, and the need to focus on anxiety as the core problem must be adhered to diligently.

DSM-5 AND CHAPTER 19

DISSOCIATIVE, SOMATOFORM, AND FACTITIOUS DISORDERS

Somatic Symptom Disorder is now an umbrella term that combines several previous somatoform disorders such as Hypochondriasis and Somatization Disorder into one broader category. A problem in DSM-IV was overlap and a lack of clear boundaries among the somatoform diagnoses.

Those who have complex medical problems with psychiatric features can be addressed with this diagnosis. The previous requirement for at least 6 months of unexplained medical symptoms has been dropped under DSM-5. A disproportionate or maladaptive concern by an individual for his or her symptoms can now be taken into consideration in establishing this diagnosis.

Challenges to Clinical Practice

Somatic Symptom Disorder is a diagnotic category that may be filled with people who have serious medical problems that are difficult to treat effectively. The variation in physical sensitivity to pain and the expression of disability could be interpreted as a psychiatric symptom instead of a physiological variable that exists among people. People who have complex medical problems and cannot get satisfactory help from health care providers may now be given a psychiatric diagnosis as a result. This could abbreviate or even eliminate medical interventions, and shunt clients of sub-par medical clinicians to psychiatric clinicians for treatment. Substantial numbers of people who have cancer, heart disease, diabetes, fibromyalgia, lupus, and so on—and who, in fact, have no real mental disorder beyond their deep distress and depression deriving from the inability of medical doctors to help them—could now carry a psychiatric label (Frances, 2012).

 DSM-5 AND CHAPTER 20

GENDER IDENTITY AND SEXUAL DISORDERS

The criteria for and description of Pedophilia is unchanged from DSM-IV-TR, but the disorder name is now Pedophilic Disorder.

The term Gender Identity Disorder has been changed to Gender Dysphoria and is no longer in a sexual disorders section but is, rather, in a section of its own. This represents a conceptual change more in tune with what experts in this specialty have been advocating for many years by emphasizing gender incongruence rather than cross-gender identification and removing it from the realm of sexual dysfunctions. Separate sets of criteria for children and adolescents have been developed.

Challenges to Clinical Practice

There are no specific challenges to these name changes. The characteristics of pedophilic behavior are the same from the last edition of the manual to this current one.

 DSM-5 AND CHAPTER 21

EATING DISORDERS

Binge-Eating Disorder has been moved from DSM-IV-TR's Appendix B: Criteria Sets and Axes Provided for Further Study to DSM-5's Section II Diagnostic Criteria and Codes. Further study has validated the symptoms and behaviors of people with this condition as consistent with a mental disorder.

Challenges to Clinical Practice

Excessive eating beyond nutritional needs has been a hotly debated topic for many years. Is it a matter of genetics, personal strength, a medical diagnosis, or is it addictive or psychiatric in nature? The move of this diagnosis from an appendix to the diagnoses section based upon evidence from recent research places it within the realm of psychiatry.

Binge eating 12 times in 3 months is no longer considered a manifestation of overeating resulting from the easy availability of food. The challenge for mental health professionals with this change in the diagnostic and statistical manual is to re-orient themselves to thinking of this behavior as a psychiatric illness that requires psychiatric intervention (Frances, 2012).

 DSM-5 AND CHAPTER 22

PERSONALITY DISORDERS

DSM-5 maintains the categorical model and criteria for the 10 personality disorders included in DSM-IV-TR. There is some clarification of aspects of the criteria for diagnosing personality disorders, but no substantive change has been made to the criteria at this time. The removal of the multiaxial system means that personality disorders are no longer categorized as different from the major mental disorders by placement on a separate Axis (Axis II).

There was considerable debate during the revision process about the shortcomings of this current approach to personality disorders. A separate section at the back of the manual (Alternative DSM-5 Model for Personality Disorders) includes new, personality trait–specific methodology to encourage further research on how traits can be used to diagnose personality disorders in clinical practice. The alternative model includes only six personality disorders: antisocial, avoidant, borderline, narcissistic, obsessive-compulsive, and schizotypal personality disorders. It excludes avoidant, dependent, histrionic, and schizoid personality disorders. The rationale is that these behaviors may be better explained as a normal developmental stage, a result of sociocultural environment, another medical condition, another mental disorder, or the effects of a substance.

Challenges to Clinical Practice

Anticipation of the DSM-5's perspective on personality disorders had been fraught with consternation, but there was also the fragrance of a fresh perspective. Ultimately, there have been no substantive changes made to this set of diagnostics. However, there are two issues that bear discussion. The multiaxial system has been removed, placing "personality disorders" not in its own category as separate and distinct from major mental illnesses, but listing it as another major mental illness. Those of us involved in psychoeducation and treatment can see the flaw in this. There are no specific biologic treatments (pharmacology) to address a neurotransmitter imbalance as there is with schizophrenia, bipolar disorder, or depression, for example. There are psychopharmacologic treatments for some of the symptoms people with personality disorders experience when they become depressed or unstable in their perceptions; however, there is no biologic treatment that will actually change someone's personality. Listing "personality disorders" as a major mental disorder blurs the line significantly and can make the expectation of effective treatment in the short term unrealistic.

DSM-5 AND CHAPTER 25 AND 26

CHILDREN AND ADOLESCENT POPULATIONS

The DSM-5 collapses DSM-IV-TR's Pervasive Developmental Disorder (PDD) and its subtypes Autistic Disorder, Asperger's Disorder, Childhood Disintegrative Disorder, and Pervasive Developmental Disorder (Not Otherwise Specified), into the single diagnosis of Autism Spectrum Disorder. This change is intended to more accurately and consistently diagnose children with autism, assess the severity of the disorder, and identify the supports needed to treat the disorder effectively.

The diagnosis of Mental Retardation has been changed to Intellectual Disability. This reflects the use of a term in common use among medical, educational, and advocacy groups. New diagnostic criteria emphasize the need to assess adaptive functioning as well as IQ score. Severity is now determined by adaptive functioning rather than IQ score.

DSM-5 also broadens the criteria for learning disorders to represent distinct disorders that interfere with language acquisition and the use of oral language, reading, writing, or mathematics, or a combination of these. Specific learning-disorders criteria are more inclusive and demonstrate sensitivity to the myriad manners of expression of disability or lessened ability.

Disruptive Mood Dysregulation Disorder is a new diagnosis included in DSM-5 to diagnose children who exhibit persistent irritability and frequent episodes of behavioral or verbal outbursts three or more times a week for more than a year. The diagnosis is intended to address concerns about potential overdiagnosis and overtreatment of bipolar disorder in children.

The revised PTSD diagnostic criteria are more developmentally sensitive and specific for children and adolescents.

Challenges to Clinical Practice

The definition of autism, once employed, can result in lower rates of the diagnosis. The criteria change may enhance our accuracy and specificity; however, there could be an unintended disruptive influence. The potential for fewer diagnoses of autism in children would also mean a lesser investment in school services, treatment provision, and family assistance. The challenge could be in helping families of autism-spectrum children maintain intact mental health service delivery.

Regarding the new diagnosis Disruptive Mood Dysregulation Disorder, a treatment challenge could be whether to medicate children diagnosed with this new label. Verbal outbursts and temper tantrums could be interpreted as a mental disorder. If so, would this lead to medicating more young children rather than providing behavioral programs? As one clinician suggests (Frances, 2012), it is difficult to accurately diagnose children and avoid the risks of overmedicating them. He believes that DSM-5 should not have added a new disorder likely to result in a new fad and even more inappropriate medication use in vulnerable children.

Changing the term Mental Retardation to Intellectual Disability has been a "long time coming." DSM-IV had been out-of-sync with educators, advocacy groups, and lay people for some time.